METASTATIC BREAST CANCER:
FROM DIAGNOSIS TO COMPLETE REMISSION

An Intentional Journey

DENICE JEFFERY

For book orders, email orders@traffordpublishing.com.sg

Most Trafford Singapore titles are also available at major online book retailers.

© Copyright 2012 Denice Jeffery.
All rights reserved. No part of this publication may be reproduced, stored in a retrieval system, or transmitted, in any form or by any means, electronic, mechanical, photocopying, recording, or otherwise, without the written prior permission of the author.

This is what worked for me. You should consult your health practitioners before starting on a regime of supplementation.

Printed in Singapore.

ISBN: 978-1-4669-3127-5 (sc)
ISBN: 978-1-4669-3128-2 (hc)
ISBN: 978-1-4669-3129-9 (e)

Trafford rev. 11/05/2012

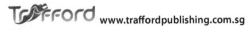 www.traffordpublishing.com.sg

Singapore
toll-free: 800 101 2656 (Singapore)
Fax: 800 101 2656 (Singapore)

DEDICATION

In memory of my cousin Ian, a beautiful man, taken too early—thank you for starting with me and supporting me on my journey.

Thanks to my husband Bill and my family, in particular, Helen—without your love and support, I could not have done this, and no doubt, I would not be here.

And finally, for my friend Jean, with love, hope, and faith—I believe you can do this too.

PREFACE

Life! It seems sometimes that the old cliché is true; it can change in an instant.

One minute, I had a very painful shoulder. The next, the doctor had placed a radiology report under my nose and said 'Here, read this . . . ' Two little words, which instil a feeling of terror, dread, and overwhelming uncertainty and which will continue to resonate indefinitely, stick in my mind: 'multiple metastases'. Life changed at that moment, and our nightmarish, emotional rollercoaster ride began.

Why write a book? There are a few reasons: I found it difficult and frustrating navigating the Internet for information. I wanted information fast, and while there is a plethora of information on the Internet, a lot of it is conflicting. I also wasn't aware that bone metastases were common after breast cancer, and women need to be aware that it can happen. Furthermore, it does not necessarily mean a death sentence as suggested by my doctors, and there is hope. Lastly, it is possible that some health professionals may not only learn from the 'account of my illness' narrative, but I am hoping it may also increase their awareness and insight.

So I am hoping this book will provide information and useful websites, and increase awareness of bone metastases. I'm also hoping that this will inspire those with cancer to make some changes and live a long, full, and healthy life.

This book is about my journey and what worked for me. It is not meant to replace medical advice, but rather, it is meant to provide information and education. Much of this book represents my opinion. Given that cancer is complex and each individual is different, this information should not be viewed as an authority on cancer treatment, but more as an unsubstantiated literary work which obviously has not been reviewed by our Therapeutic Goods Administration. What worked for me is integrative treatment, and I believe that many people are now looking for this and probably feeling as frustrated as I am that some doctors are ignorant when it comes to nutrition and complementary therapies. Some oncologists and doctors are just not interested in anything outside their medical paradigm, and this too I found very frustrating.

This book is divided into two parts. The first part is my story, and the second part lists the strategies, protocols, and supplements that I utilised in detail, along with website links.

Note: Before embarking on any programme of supplementation or changes to dietary regimes, it is strongly recommended that health professionals, such as doctors, naturopaths, oncology pharmacists, and others be consulted initially as some supplements and strategies may be contraindicated.

Cancer, even late stage, does not have to be a death sentence.

(Robert Jay Rowen in *Defeat Cancer* by Connie Strasheim,
Biomed Publishing Group, 2011)

PART 1
MY STORY

CHAPTER 1

My journey began five years earlier in 2005. I had noticed a dimple on my right breast and knew that there was a very good possibility that I had cancer as one of my elder sisters had been diagnosed a few years before at the same age of forty-six.

We have a strong family history of breast cancer. My mother's mother had a double mastectomy due to breast cancer, and her sister died from it. My mother's paternal grandmother died from breast cancer at the age of fifty-three. My paternal aunt had breast cancer, and another aunt ovarian cancer. My cousin had prostate cancer. My own mother had eight children and two miscarriages and had been pregnant or breastfeeding for about seventeen years. In other words, she was not exposed to the same risk as me as I could not have children.

After my mammogram in 2005, I was told that I had to wait for two weeks for the films to be read, and apparently, this was not uncommon in Cairns. I was told by the nurse at the breast clinic that 'in the scheme of things, two weeks would not make any difference'. Well, I disagreed. In my line of work as a psychologist, I have to deal with my issues quickly. How could I concentrate on my work and my clients' issues if I was facing a huge issue myself? I rang a clinic in Brisbane, 1,700 km away, and asked if the films could be seen there. I was seen a few days later, and on the same day, I had a biopsy which confirmed early breast cancer. It was exactly the same type as my sister's three years earlier.

While I was on the table having my biopsy, I remember thinking about my poodle puppy, Penne, and smiling. She had been a gift from my husband a few weeks earlier. I saw her in a pet shop, something I usually avoided, and it was love at first sight. I told my husband about her and told him that she was too expensive and that we couldn't afford her. That night, I dreamt of her and told him the next morning. The day after I saw her in the pet shop, I came home from work, and she met me at the door. She was meant to be. She is still with me, and now has a little mate—another poodle called Miss Poppy.

I saw the breast surgeon and had a lumpectomy a couple of weeks later. His report noted that 'margins were close'. He suggested that the cancer had been there for at least five years—it seems it had been missed by the radiologists for a few years.

I then had to wait for eleven weeks for radiation due to waiting times, a situation which is totally unacceptable in terms of best practice. We had to travel from Cairns to Townsville, a distance of about 400 km, for treatment, and I nearly gave up in despair as I couldn't initially find accommodation that would take Penne, another source of distress. Eventually, the Cancer Council found us a unit, which allowed us to take her. I wasn't going anywhere without her. My poodles have been a constant source of love and joy throughout my journey.

I had regular blood tests for the next five years. In March 2008, my husband was made redundant from his job, and I became the sole income earner. In May 2008, I had a bone scan which was all clear. In July, my husband came to work with me in my office, and I started to work longer hours. In August that year, my right shoulder became painful, and I saw three doctors over a period of time and had two ultrasounds.

These revealed a slight tear of my tendon. My shoulder didn't improve, and I couldn't do anything with it. I couldn't use it to clean or swim or dig in the garden without suffering severe, debilitating pain. I put off seeing a sports doctor, my fourth, about my shoulder because I was 'too busy' at work. I didn't make time for my health and only saw another doctor about my shoulder in January 2010, about eighteen months after it first became painful. He referred me urgently to an orthopaedic surgeon, who requested an MRI. I suspect the sports doctor, unlike the other three I had seen, knew exactly what he was dealing with, given my history of breast cancer.

Take-Home Messages

1. When undergoing unpleasant procedures, focus on something or someone that gives you love and joy.
2. If you choose to have radiation, don't wait as long as I did. Talk to your doctors about ideal waiting times.
3. Take control. If you have to wait for results, see what else can be done to minimise waiting times.
4. A breast cancer diagnosis does not necessarily mean a death sentence.
5. Health always comes first before work. Reassess your values and prioritise them. You cannot work if you don't have your health.
6. If you don't get satisfaction from one doctor, see another. Get a second, third, and fourth opinion if you must.
7. If you have pain in any area which persists after a breast cancer diagnosis, insist on appropriate tests, MRIs, specialist referrals, and so on. Don't ignore it and hope that it will go away.
8. Identify what stressors you have been subjected to six to eighteen months prior to the onset of the cancer. What changes have taken place during this time? The onset of cancer may well suggest that you are not able to cope effectively with those changes. Have you had any other

illnesses, and if so, did any particular stressful event precede it or them?
9. Useful websites include the following:

   a. http://canceraustralia.nbocc.org.au/risk/riskfactors.html
   b. http://www.ranzcr.edu.au/quality-a-safety/radiation-oncology

We must look for the causes of disease and deal with those, rather than focus solely on symptom management, an unfortunate reality of pharmaceutical based medicine.

(Richard Linchitz, MD, in *Defeat Cancer* by Connie Strasheim, Biomed Publishing Group, 2011)

CHAPTER 2

Individuals respond differently to the same news. When I got the news of my metastases, I went into shock. This wasn't supposed to happen to me—it happens to other people. My five-year anniversary (from the time of initial diagnosis) was just around the corner. It took a few hours to sink in.

My husband, on the other hand, became emotional and upset immediately. He spoke to the doctor in private, and to this day, I don't know what about. I do know he got a script for some sleeping pills.

We walked away from the surgery, not knowing what kind of metastases I had, where they were, what my prognosis was, or even if I had a future. If you think a breast cancer diagnosis is scary, imagine that fear multiplied many, many times over, and you may come close to experiencing the feeling of terror instilled by those two little words—'multiple metastases'.

We made it home somehow, and by this time, the news was starting to sink in. I was sick to my stomach. Anxiety was sky high, and not having information made it worse. My sister Kate and her husband arrived, and we broke the news to them. I wasn't sure I would survive.

We made it through the next several days. My husband and I watched the entire series of *Battlestar Galactica* during these weeks, and to this day, I associate it with this particular period of my life—rather unpleasant. We had to wait a week for an appointment to see my breast surgeon. In the meantime, I had a bone scan, which revealed several bone metastases from my head to my pelvis. A subsequent CT scan revealed a spot on my lung, which was reported as 7 cm, but which turned out to be a typo—it was 7 mm. I also had a positive node in my neck. My breast surgeon told me that it would 'take me out' within five to ten years. I had been given a terminal diagnosis.

The waiting continued, as I waited a few weeks to see the oncologist at the hospital. My breast surgeon, a man with many years' experience with cancer patients and one I trust, had already suggested a possible treatment plan, and this was confirmed by the oncologist. Monthly, Zometa IV, a bisphosphonate, and Zoladex injections to switch off my ovaries and Arimidex, an aromatase inhibitor, were administered. I refused to take Tamoxifen™ because of previous research, and this is another story.

In the middle of all this, I got the flu which I had for several weeks. I had time off work to deal with the flu and the diagnosis. I became anaemic and needed blood transfusions. Luckily for me, I didn't realise how sick I was at the time.

I knew I didn't want to die. I couldn't do that to my family. I also knew that if I depended on medicine for a cure, I wasn't going to get one. Mainstream medicine concentrates on 'evidence-based science', which suggests rigorous studies, although some people may disagree. The gold standard study is a double-blind, placebo-controlled trial involving many people. Researchers look for statistically significant results, and the drugs which achieve these results become valid options for medical treatment. Results which have been documented by medical practitioners based on the observations they achieved with their patients are generally known as 'anecdotal evidence'. Most private practitioners cannot afford to conduct the gold standard clinical trial, and only pharmaceutical companies can generally afford these, hence the paucity of evidence-based material relative to alternative medicine.

I had been told by my doctors that there was no cure; it was terminal. I chose not to believe them, and Dr Jenkins from the Budwig Cancer Centre confirmed this belief. I was also told by a friend's husband, a doctor, to focus on 'surviving' and not to worry about a cure. This was never good enough for me. I became obsessive. I was determined to become a conundrum to my oncologist, and my aim was to be able to say to her, 'Neener, neener, neener, (told you so)'—childish, I know, but the thought of it gave me enormous pleasure and inspiration.

Take-Home Messages

1. Have a purpose—focus on it. Become determined, focus on the future you want for yourself. Have a reason for living.
2. What are your beliefs about life? What you believe about life will influence your desire to live. For example, if you love life and believe life to be good, you will want to live.
3. Keep busy while you are waiting and don't have all the information. When you start to catastrophise, tell yourself to 'stop', and get yourself distracted. Do deep breathing to calm yourself. Don't be afraid to ask your doctor for sleeping pills or a sedative, as I believe they have a part to play in this situation.
4. Come up with a long list of enjoyable activities to do, and make sure you do at least one each day.
5. Individuals respond differently to a cancer diagnosis. Responses range from mild to severe. Some people cope better than others. Coping isn't static, that is, some days may be better than others. Some may develop anxiety or depression, and these feelings too can also come and go. One in four cancer patients become depressed. Signs that someone is

not adjusting include a loss of interest in previously enjoyed activities and a loss of pleasure or joy. These must persist for a minimum of two weeks to meet the criteria of a depressive disorder. If you have difficulty adjusting to a cancer diagnosis, consider a consultation with a psychologist.
6. Sadness and grief are normal reactions to a cancer diagnosis.
7. Finding out about cancer can result in feelings of disbelief, denial, or despair. I went into shock. Sleeping difficulties, loss of appetite, anxiety, and some depressed mood may also be experienced. As the cancer patient adjusts, the symptoms may improve. Signs of adjustment include an ability to maintain daily activities, an ability to continue functioning as a spouse, parent, employee, or other roles, and by incorporating treatment into the cancer patient's usual regime.
8. The types of issues a cancer patient can confront include fear of death, changes to life plans, pain, financial issues, treatment decisions and related issues, changes in body image and self-esteem, work, and changes in social role and lifestyle.
9. Consider medical marijuana—this can be excellent for coping with anxiety as well as pain and also very useful for enhancing sleep for some. This is something that I have recently been reading about, and it is a pity that I found out about it at this time and not sooner. The Internet abounds with anecdotal stories about people who have not only used cannabis to assist with symptom management, but there are also stories about people who have used it to overcome their cancer.

The greatest healers have been great healers precisely because of their ability to influence their patients' expectations and beliefs.

(Richard Linchitz, MD, in *Defeat Cancer* by Connie Strasheim, Biomed Publishing Group, 2011)

CHAPTER 3

While I had the flu and had time off work, I started to read. One book in particular by Deepak Chopra (*Reinventing the Body, Resurrecting the Soul*) contained advice which I believe served me well—acting with intention is everything. I got it—I intended to be well, and I had to behave with intention. But, where to start with the diet? I knew from what I had read that diet was important. What else did I need to do? I continued to read. The Internet is replete with information and a lot of it is conflicting. I knew from my reading that I had to treat myself holistically, which meant that I had to sort my issues, develop spiritually, and take care of myself physically.

I read *The Power of Now* by Eckhart Tolle, a book I had bought a few years earlier and wasn't ready for. I was this time. I learned to live in the present.

I also read a book called *The Journey* by Brandon Bays. I did the processes outlined in the book and sorted my long-standing issues. I cried and cried, and my husband was there for comfort at the end of each session. The book outlines a process for getting to the 'source' as she calls it, and it worked for me. For the first time in my life, I not only knew I was loved, but I felt loved, and I felt worthwhile. I experienced sheer joy, an overwhelming sense of love, and peace, and I learned to go there repeatedly in just a few minutes. It was an incredible, cathartic experience and something I will encourage everyone to do.

I read Carl Simonton's books (listed below) and took myself through the processes outlined in his books. I listened to his CDs. These are worthwhile, and they are highly recommended. I visualised, breathed, meditated, and relaxed.

I read whatever I could find on the Internet about cancer and remedies—mainly accessing alternative sites. I read about alkalising and how cancer can't survive in a pH of 8.5. How this is known is beyond me. I read that cancer loves an acidic body, and found alkaway.com, where I ordered alkalising drops for my water. I read about earthing, sunshine, deep breathing, and all sorts of supplements. I also found e-books on alternative cancer clinics in Germany and Mexico, and these became my plan B.

Take-Home Messages

1. Become informed about diet and dietary supplements. Read books which help you to come to terms with your emotional issues and which help you develop spiritually. Take responsibility for your health and actively participate in your own healing process.
2. Become aware of your thoughts and any negative feelings, such as resentment, anger, blame, and failure. Become responsible for your own happiness as well as your health. Learn to express emotions in a healthy way. Concentrate your thoughts on things that are uplifting. Surround yourself with supportive people.
3. Have a plan A and a plan B. Plan A was doing this by myself, and plan B was an alternative cancer clinic in Germany. This gave me a heightened sense of control. Plan C, my last resort, was chemo as I had read in many places on the Internet that chemo only helps about 3 per cent of people. Furthermore, I couldn't do chemo because my white cell count and

neutrophils were really low. Chemo also affects all cells, not just cancer cells.

4. Books I found helpful include the following:

   a. *The Power of Now* by Eckhart Tolle
   b. *The Journey* by Brandon Bays
   c. *Reinventing the Body, Resurrecting the Soul* by Deepak Chopra
   d. *The Healing Journey* by O. Carl Simonton, MD, and his CD *Getting Well*
   e. *Dietary Healing* by Kathryn Alexander

5. Learn to meditate. Read *The Healing Journey*, and do the meditations in the book.

6. When feeling overwhelmed, close your eyes and listen to the sounds all around you—focus on them for a few minutes and give your mind a break. Open your heart with compassion to others—send good vibes to those undergoing cancer treatment or those suffering ill health. This may help reduce those feelings of loneliness and connect you to others. Another tip when feeling anxious is to imagine a place that you love and where you feel at peace and then go there in your mind. Imagine the sight, sound, and smell of the place. Stay there until you are calm. Repeat affirmations such as 'I can do this' or make up your own affirmation, one that works for you. Try deep breathing—in through your nose and out through your mouth. Count down from ten to one. Breathe slowly and deeply and notice it relaxing your body. Finally, find some things to be grateful for—this can be difficult; however, I found many things, including my family, my poodles, my garden, the sun, flowers, and so on. This does help to lift the mood, and it also helps to make this a daily habit if you can.

7. The acid and alkaline chart will give you an idea of what foods belong in which category. There is lots of information about this on the Internet.
8. Useful websites include the following

    a. http://www.cancertutor.com
    b. http://www.imva.com
    c. http://www.ralphmoss.com
    d. http://www.beating-cancer-gently.com/
    e. http://www.budwigcenter.com/
    f. http://www.mskcc.org/cancer-care/integrative-medicine/about-herbs
    g. http://health.groups.yahoo.com/group/iodine/
    h. http://breastcancerchoices.org/iprotocol.html
    i. http://www.germancancerclinics.com/
    j. http://www.cancure.org/directory_mexican_clinics.htm
    k. http://www.beyondblue.org.au/index.aspx?
    l. http://www.cancer.gov/cancertopics/coping
    m. http://www.cancer.org/Treatment/TreatmentsandSideEffects/ComplementaryandAlternativeMedicine/guidelines-for-using-complementary-and-alternative-methods
    n. http://www.mexicancancerclinics.com/?gclid=CPjejYiEw7ICFXBUpgodCkoAMw

A Canadian survey of oncologists found that few oncologists, if any, would take their own potions.

20 % of many cancers are destined to go nowhere even if not treated at all.

(Robert Jay Rowen, MD, in *Defeat Cancer* by Connie Strasheim, Biomed Publishing Group, 2011)

CHAPTER 4

My husband, who had been working with me, left to work overseas as he needed to provide financial support, and I was on my own. I realised that being on my own was not a good idea as I had too much time to ruminate. I did not need to focus on the cancer or my doctor's grim prognosis that it would take me out. I had one really bad night after I read a website which scared the hell out of me. I had a session with my supervisor, a psychiatrist, who wrote me a script for an anti-psychotic, which would knock me out if I needed it. As I never had another bad night, I never got the script filled.

My cousin Ian, who had been diagnosed with prostate cancer many years before and was then diagnosed with mesothelioma, came to stay for a few weeks with his daughter Nell and her husband Eli in July 2010. He suggested Bill Henderson's e-book, and we both devoured and discussed it. We became cancer buddies and the Henderson protocol became plan A.

We started on a gluten-free, mostly dairy-free, sugar-free, alcohol-free, caffeine-free, organic, vegetarian diet. We also started on Budwig smoothies—a blend of quark (this was the only dairy in the diet) and flaxseed oil along with almond milk, berries, and banana. I knew after a week of drinking the smoothie that something had changed for the better for me as my breathing had improved. I had been unable to take a breath without it catching, and this stopped. It was at this time that I realised I had to give up dairy—another message from Deepak Chopra—listen to your body. I was sick of the coughing associated with it. I think I am probably lactose intolerant. The only dairy I continued to eat was the quark in the smoothie.

I reintroduced some organic meat after my visitors left as I needed protein and wasn't sure I was getting enough. I started on the supplements recommended by Bill Henderson. I knew from what I had read that good nutrition is important, so I started to drink BarleyLife, Just Carrots, and RediBeets. I bought the dried products from AIM, a wholefood nutrition company (website given below), rather than make my own. I had a glass of BarleyLife 3 times a day before meals and one glass of Just Carrots and RediBeets every day.

A few weeks after Ian left, I realised, thanks to a friend, that I needed support. One phone call and my sister Helen arrived shortly after to stay for the next twelve months while my husband worked overseas. I will be forever grateful to my sister and my parents for the gift of a big family.

Take-Home Messages

1. Having support is crucial. This is especially true when you visit with doctors. It helps to have another person present to remember to ask questions and to listen as well. The other person can even take notes.
2. Ask for help. Don't assume that others know what you need.
3. It is helpful if you can have a cancer buddy, someone to support you, and to help you research.
4. If you don't have time or can't afford lots of organic vegetables, then drink the AIM products. Their website is http://www.theaimcompanies.com/
5. Flood your body with good nutrition.
6. I ate some organic meat, and this did not appear to affect my recovery. I assume it is therefore acceptable. The protein

chart will give you an idea of how much protein is in certain foods.
7. Adopt a gluten-free, dairy-free, sugar-free, alcohol-free, caffeine-free, organic, mostly vegetarian diet.
8. Drink the Budwig smoothie at least once every day. Watch how it is made here http://www.johanabudwig.com/
9. Check with your doctor before starting the smoothie. I started on four tablespoons of flaxseed oil per day, and I did this for a month before cutting down to ½-2 tablespoons daily. If you have liver issues, you may have to start with way less—do your research and consult a health practitioner. I used flaxseed oil as this is what Johanna Budwig recommended, and this is what her research was based on.
10. Be aware that tablespoon measures vary from country to country. The Australian tablespoon is 20 ml and the American tablespoon is about 15 ml.
11. What are the secondary gains of your cancer? Mine was having my sister with me, taking care of me and also lots of attention from my family.
12. How does cancer help you to cope with stress? Does it allow you to say 'no', for example? Does it allow you to say 'yes' to important parts of yourself that you may have previously denied? I allowed myself to sit on the couch and snuggle my poodles.
13. Has cancer given you the freedom to focus on your life in a different way?
14. Cancer can be a message to stop doing things that cause you pain.
15. Bill Henderson's website is http://www.beating-cancer-gently.com/
16. Check out websites such as this one given below to see what organic foods you need to buy:

a) http://greenopolis.com/myopolis/blogs/aresende/what-you-should-shouldnt-buy-organic; or
b) http://www.eatingwell.com/food_news_origins/organic_natural/15_foods_you_dont_need_to_buy_organic
c) http://www.ewg.org/foodnews/list/

I've had several patients go into remission with just diet, supplements, and detoxification strategies. But cancer is a lifelong treatment.

(Robert Jay Rowen, MD, in *Defeat Cancer* by Connie Strasheim, Biomed Publishing Group, 2011)

CHAPTER 5

I stayed on Bill Henderson's protocol all the time, continuing to read about alternative cancer treatments and working part time. I continued to read about cancer centres, supplements, and alkalising. I became frustrated that a lot of the supplements that were touted as cancer cures did not have an evidence base. Some of the protocols did not have any science at all behind them, just lots of testimonials and anecdotal stories. Navigating through all the information was time-consuming, frustrating, and tricky. I found a good starting point for research was the Sloan Kettering herbs website.

In June 2010, I had a week of radiation, with massive doses to three areas. My scapula, spine, and pelvis were all treated. We had to travel to Townsville once again as radiation was not available in Cairns. If I knew then what I know now, I would have declined to have radiation. I experienced my very first panic attack on the radiation table, and I think at some level I knew I was getting too much. The radiation went on for what seemed to be such a long time that I panicked. I devised a strategy to ensure that I would cope with further radiation sessions. I asked the radiation therapist to let me know how long each session would last, and then I counted down until it was over. With this strategy and deep breathing, I managed each session.

After the week of intensive radiation, I developed neutropenia and pancytopenia, that is, low white cells, low red cells, and low platelets. I had a 'bone marrow' response to the radiation. No information was given to me by anyone as to how to cope with this. I have since found that there is information on the Internet about what type of diet is best suited to neutropenia, and the link is given below.

I researched 'bone marrow' on the Sloan Kettering website and came up with some supplements that I could take to support my bone marrow. I started to take Maitake and Melatonin. Bill Henderson also suggests that Transfer Point's Beta Glucan can benefit the bone marrow, and I have taken this on and off.

My health slowly improved over several months. My haemoglobin eventually came good, and I no longer needed the transfusions I had been having. My tumour marker returned to 'normal', but after a few months, it began to climb slightly. I had tumour marker tests done every two months, and the days before I got my result, I was filled with anxiety and the 'what ifs'. I asked for and kept copies of all my blood tests results in a folder so I could keep track of my results and look for trends. Keeping busy while waiting for blood test results became the norm.

When I was having my blood tests including tumour marker tests, I initially alternated between the hospital and a private laboratory. My tumour marker varied quite widely, and it took some months before I ascertained that something was amiss, and in fact, the laboratories were using different tests.

Whenever I found myself starting to have doubts, or my anxiety increased, I found that reading stories on the Internet of people who have survived cancer did two things. It alleviated my anxiety and provided me with an inspirational and motivational boost. The Internet is full of stories of people who have beaten cancer in every stage.

In December 2010, I had a PET/CT scan. I knew from what I had read that only a PET/CT could tell the difference between a lysing (dying) tumour and a live one. My oncologist said that the results revealed that my tumours were 'getting worse'. I assume this meant that they were either getting bigger or they had become more active. Anyhow, my response to this was 'I don't think so'. I felt better, not worse. She suggested chemo, but I declined. My neutrophils were in the very low range of normal, slightly above the cut off point for chemo. I didn't think I would survive the chemo. I contacted my breast surgeon who agreed with me. Just because the CT scan suggested an increase in activity did not necessarily mean the tumours were getting worse. Looking back now, I'm wondering if they were indeed lysing then, and the CT scan picked this up and represented it as 'increased activity'. I suspect that in all probability, the Henderson protocol was working.

Take-Home Messages

1. Listen to your body.
2. Just because a CT scan shows 'increased activity' does not necessarily mean that tumours are getting worse.
3. Don't forget, you and your oncologist are in this together. You can choose to make collaborative decisions. Doctors are trained in the prevailing belief system of their profession. If you have a doctor with a negative attitude, you can view this as their beliefs, *not* yours. Detach. If you can do this, you need not be overwhelmed by their authority and can be more objective about the treatment and care you are receiving. This is crucial if your doctor has no regard for your attitude towards healing or getting well. You can make a list of beliefs about your doctor and evaluate how healthy these beliefs are. Keep the healthy ones and discard or change the unhealthy ones.
4. Don't be afraid to get a second opinion or a third opinion.

5. A PET/CT can give useful information and can also distinguish between live and dead or dying tumours. It is helpful to have one of these early so that a baseline may be established and used for comparison as treatment progresses. A CT scan does not give the same useful information.
6. There is lots of conflicting information on the Internet about remedies. Use your instinct to go with what is best for you. Talk to others. A lot of remedies are not evidence based, something which I found very frustrating. Check out the website given below (b) for some guidelines.
7. If you choose to have radiation, check out possible side effects first to ensure you are fully informed.
8. Ask for copies of your blood test results and watch for trends. This helps with a feeling of empowerment.
9. Be aware that not all pathology laboratories use the same tests for tumour markers—once you have a tumour marker done, continue to go back to the same lab.
10. Useful websites include the following:

    a. http://www.radiologyinfo.org/en/info.cfm?pg=pet
    b. http://www.cancer.org/Treatment/TreatmentsandSideEffects/ComplementaryandAlternativeMedicine/guidelines-for-using-complementary-and-alternative-methods
    c. http://www.mskcc.org/cancer-care/integrative-medicine/about-herbs
    d. http://www.nhlcyberfamily.org/treatments/neutropenic.htm
    e. http://www.betterhealth.vic.gov.au/bhcv2/bhcarticles.nsf/pages/Cancer_treatments_radiotherapy
    f. http://oncologygroupassignmentsp2011.wikispaces.com/Anemia,+neutropenia,+thrombocytopenia,+and+pancytopenia

g. http://inhealth.about.com/when-cancer-care-leads-to-neutropenia/diet-dos-and-donts-with-neutropenia?did=t5_rss38
h. http://inhealth.cnn.com/when-cancer-care-leads-to-neutropenia/

Cancer cells are actually, weak, deformed, and confused. No cancer cell has ever been shown to attack a healthy cell. Cancer can't even grow very well inside a strong, healthy body. Cancer can only thrive inside a weakened, unhealthy body. It's that simple.

(Carl O. Simonton in *Cancer Breakthrough USA—A Guide to Outstanding Alternative Clinics* by Frank Cousineau with Andrew Scholberg, Online Publishing and Marketing LLC, 2009)

CHAPTER 6

In early 2011, I discovered a distance programme offered by a cancer centre in Spain—the Budwig cancer centre. I knew from my reading that it was best to stick with a protocol and given I had faith in the Budwig smoothie, I contacted them. I started on their programme in July 2011. I had been on the Henderson protocol for about twelve months at this stage.

I had also read e-books written by Mark Sircus on sodium bicarbonate (bicarb), magnesium, and cancer. Mark suggests that every person with a chronic illness is deficient in magnesium, so I started using transdermal magnesium as well as oral magnesium chloride. I also read the story of Vernon at phkillscancer.com and decided to try his remedy of bicarb and blackstrap molasses. Over the months, I did that protocol several times. I think it worked because when I was having the Zometa IV, my bone metastases would burn at times. Looking back now, I'm not sure it was the right thing to do. What happens when acid meets bicarb? It fizzes, and perhaps this explains the burning sensation in my bones . . . No one could tell me any information, and I had to wing it.

In April 2011, I had my last Zometa IV. I had an atypical fracture on my left wrist and pain in my jaw on both sides—both possible side effects of the Zometa. I was not offered an X-ray for my wrist; although, I complained to all doctors. I should have requested one. I decided to listen to my body—no more Zometa. My oncologist and breast surgeon weren't happy, but I didn't need their approval.

Take-Home Messages

1. Listen to your body.
2. If you decide to make a decision about treatment, you don't necessarily need to have your treating doctor's approval. Sometimes, we do know what we need best.
3. If you decide to try the bicarb-molasses protocol, you need to check with your doctor first. There may well be some contraindications, for example, if you have kidney problems. You can also have a skype consultation with Mark Sircus from imva.com, and he can guide you through it.
4. It may be necessary sometimes to ask your doctors for specific tests or X-rays. All they can say is 'No'.
5. Useful websites include the following:

    a. http://phkillscancer.com/
    b. http://www.budwigcenter.com/
    c. http://imva.info/

My overall treatment philosophy for cancer is to trap the cancer in a deadly crossfire and beat the crap out of it with safe concentrated nutritional medicinals and solid health practices including plenty of sun exposure, exercise, touch via massage, and breathing techniques that you can see on Vernon's site. But, as Vernon's case demonstrates, the sodium bicarbonate is the lead Panzer Division that has the power to kick ass pretty much all by itself . . . Same can be said of iodine and magnesium chloride.

(Mark Sircus at http://imva.info/index.php/2009/10/still-alive-and-well/)

CHAPTER 7

In May 2011, the constant, severe pain in my wrist was affecting my sleep. Further research led me to pulse emitted magnetic field therapy (PEMF). I purchased an MRS 2000 online, and it was here in July. I started using it three times a day, and within a few months, my wrist pain had diminished. I started to treat my bone metastases in October twice per day for eight minutes each time. I used it for three hours per day every day for six months. PEMF has Federal Drug Administration (FDA) approval for bone density, as well as pain management. It also seems to have a beneficial effect on mood and sleep. My poodles kept me company on the body mat when I was treating myself, and every day I was in fits of laughter, as my white one, Penne, had her ways and means of ensuring that she was continuously stroked. She has this habit of going straight for my ears if I stopped, so she had me trained well. I think she thought that this was her time. Everything I was doing was with the intention of getting well.

In 2009, I had a bone density scan which revealed pre-osteoporotic hips. Both the drugs I continued to take, Zoladex and Arimidex, adversely affect bone density, so I knew I had to keep up the PEMF mat if I didn't want fractures. I also had to take calcium, but having read Mark Sircus's books, I also knew that magnesium as well as vitamin D_3 was important for strong bones. I later read about elemental calcium and how it appears that it can cause heart problems.

I have since learned that a recent study found that bisphosphonate drugs such as Zometa have been found to significantly increase the risk of atypical bone fractures, the longer the drug is taken. The risk was found to be increased in a linear fashion. For example, those taking bisphosphonates for less than two years were thirty-five times more likely to have an atypical bone fracture. Those who took the medication for two to five years experience a forty-seven-fold increase in atypical fractures and so on. The link is at (h) given below.

Take-Home Messages

1. Pulse emitted magnetic field therapy has been approved by the Federal Drug Administration (FDA) in the United States for bone density and pain management. I also found it useful for maintaining mood and, initially, to help me sleep. It healed my wrist, and many studies have been done which confirms it's efficacy in treating un-united fractures.
2. Avoid elemental calcium. Refer to the link (d) given below and in the chart at page 79 to compare calcium products. The chart identifies non-dairy sources of calcium.
3. Mark Sircus recommends magnesium chloride, both oral and transdermal. He suggests that everyone with a chronic illness is magnesium deficient. To increase levels quickly, he suggests a transdermal application because if we take too much magnesium orally, it may not be absorbed. With a low magnesium intake, calcium goes out of the bones to increase the calcium levels in tissues, while a high-magnesium intake causes calcium to go out of the tissues and into the bones. A list of magnesium-rich foods can be found at the link (e) given below and in the chart at page 78.
4. If you are prescribed bisphosphonates, discuss the risks with your doctor.

5. Useful websites include the following:

    a. http://www.pemft.com/
    b. http://www.imva.com
    c. http://saveourbones.com/calcium-heart-attack/
    d. http://www.algaecal.com/supplement-comparisons/best-calcium-supplement.html
    e. http://www.algaecal.com/magnesium/magnesium-rich-foods.html
    f. http://www.naturalnews.com/036042_biphosphonate_osteoporosis_bone_fractures.html
    g. http://www.medicalnewstoday.com/articles/245762.php
    h. http://drdavidbrownstein.blogspot.com.au/2012/05/another-nail-in-coffin-for-bisphonate.html

... Never take defeat. When all is lost, try something new. Life is too precious to let it slip away from lack of initiative or plain inertia.

(Hulda R. Clark, Ph.D., ND, in *The Cure for All Advanced Cancers*, New Century Press, 1993)

CHAPTER 8

I also read David Brownstein's book about iodine. I started iodine therapy, despite not having anyone to guide me. I couldn't find any health professionals here who knew anything about iodine supplementation; although, I eventually found a Yahoo! Group and then the Facebook group, and through them, I had a skype consultation with a naturopath in Canada who specialises in iodine use. I was warned by some health professionals that a high iodine intake would 'switch off' my thyroid.

Brownstein suggests that iodine downregulates oestrogen receptors in the breast and improves fibrocystic breast disease, a precursor to breast cancer. He also suggests that at 50 mg and above, it induces programmed cell death (apoptosis) in cancer cells. I thought it was really important to me, so I persisted. To my surprise, my fibrocystic breast condition improved. When I stopped iodine therapy, however, it returned. To this day, I continue to take 50-mg iodine daily.

Fluoride was introduced to our water supply in 2011, and I found a reverse osmosis system online. I had read that fluoride takes up iodine receptors, and I wasn't going to have that. I knew pure drinking water was important, so a friend installed the system for me.

I continued on with the Budwig distance programme, and their schedule changed a few times. I stuck with the programmes. I broke out occasionally and had a glass of wine or champagne or a real cup of coffee. I bought stevia-sweetened chocolate and made gluten-free cakes sweetened with stevia so I didn't feel too deprived. I made coconut milk ice-cream and bought coconut-milk yoghurt which was thoroughly divine.

Take-Home Messages

1. According to Brownstein, we are all iodine deficient, and iodine is crucial to breast health, so investigate supplementation. Read David Brownstein's book, and join the Yahoo! group or Facebook group. Skype consultations are available with the Facebook moderator, Stephanie Buist, a naturopath from Canada, who beat thyroid cancer with iodine and who was a patient of Brownstein's. You will need to discuss this with your doctors. If you decide to do the iodine protocol, you will also need to have an iodine-loading test. If you have breast cancer, please consider the bromide test as well. You will also need to take the companion nutrients.
2. One of the companion nutrients is selenium, and not all selenium is the same. I took Se-methyl L-selenocysteine, but I have since read about another one that was used in the cure of a man with prostate cancer. This one was a selenium yeast supplement, and the link to this story is given below (j). I took supplements because the amount of selenium in food and grain depends on the amount in the soil, and it is generally accepted that our soils are relatively depleted of selenium. I took 200 mcg daily. There are recommendations about dosage in one of the links given below (g).
3. Drink pure water—don't drink tap water. You can shop online for a reverse osmosis system if you have a fluoridated water supply. I got mine from crystalquest.com.
4. Have the occasional treat. These will be much healthier if you avoid processed foods and make your own.

5. Useful websites include the following:

    a. http://www.crystalquest.com/
    b. http://www.drbrownstein.com/homePage.php
    c. http://health.groups.yahoo.com/group/iodine/
    d. https://www.facebook.com/pages/Iodine/104003789638644
    e. http://www.breastcancerchoices.org/iprotocol.html
    f. http://www.naturalnews.com/selenium.html
    g. http://www.naturalnews.com/016446.html
    h. http://www.cancer.org/Treatment/TreatmentsandSideEffects/ComplementaryandAlternativeMedicine/HerbsVitaminsandMinerals/selenium
    i. http://www.seleniumresearch.com/
    j. http://www.onecancercure.com/ONE_CANCER_CURE.html

I know many people who were told by their doctor that their late-stage or metastasised cancer was incurable, only to completely recover later by using a non-toxic, alternative approach.

(Tanya Harter Pierce in Outsmart *Your Cancer: Alternative Non-Toxic Treatments That Work* (2nd Edition), Thoughtworks Publishing, 2009)

CHAPTER 9

My sister went home in July 2011 after twelve months with me, and I was home alone again with my poodles. My husband came and went every couple of months for a few days at a time.

I stopped work at the end of February 2012. I wanted to have another PET/CT in June, and I knew I needed to focus on getting well, not on work. This was difficult, as I think most of my family have been instilled with what I call 'the great Australian Protestant work ethic' by our father—we work unless we are dead or dying. It took me a couple of months to get used to not working. I was concerned that I may get depressed, so I asked my doctor for a referral to a psychologist. I persisted with my PEMF mat, the diet, and the supplements as well as counselling.

I was having difficulty sleeping, which seemed to be exacerbated by the Zoladex. I was having up to twenty night sweats per night at times, and I was tired, lethargic, and often fell asleep while on my mat twice a day. In desperation, I asked the oncologist about anti-depressants as I had read that a low dose of Effexor could help. She responded that it works for some and not for others, and I didn't get a script. My doctor gave me scripts for sleeping pills and a sedative, and I took these a few times a week, just to ensure that I got a few reasonable nights' sleep. I dreaded going to bed at night.

As a result of poor sleep, I was having difficulty concentrating, and my memory was poor. I often forgot appointments, even though they were written in my diary. I would forget what I was looking for and constantly felt vague.

A couple of months after I gave up work, I started to feel a lot stronger physically. I still had pain, which was helped by the PEMF mat. I still had difficulty sleeping due to night sweats and insomnia but started to feel better and stronger anyhow. I started gardening again. I felt as though I could lift again. I started to lift my bigger poodle, Poppy, who weighed 12 kg, a few times a day as weightlifting therapy to help my bones. I even felt that I could lift our grandson (my step-daughter's son) and managed that a few times too. As I knew my scan was coming up, I asked my sister Helen to come again, and she arrived in May.

In June 2012, my husband arrived home for a couple of days before we were due to fly to Brisbane for my PET/CT. Once again, our anxiety levels rose. The 'what ifs' started. I wanted to have plan B in place, in case we got bad news. Germany had always been on the radar as I had been impressed by what I had read about their clinics. I found I coped better if I had plans in place.

My scan was on the Monday, and from lunchtime the day before, no carbohydrates were allowed. I found it easier this time as I had realised from my previous scan that I had been carb addicted. We returned home to Cairns on the Tuesday, and my appointment to get the result was on the Wednesday afternoon.

During the wait, anxiety levels were high. We tried to keep busy and distracted. Time seemed to slow down. Eventually, we were in the office, and the oncologist seemed to take his time with the results. He discussed my bone density, which I knew was now normal. He then looked at the PET/CT report and said that I had an 'exceptional response to endocrine therapy'. Meaning what? Meaning that the radioactive sugar solution used in the scan did not trace any cancer at all. All tumours previously identified were now 'inactive'. We were incredulous and didn't know whether to laugh or cry, so we did both. It took some time to sink in, again. I had done it—had done what I set out to do. It took me some hours to let everyone know, and the next day when the full extent of the news had sunk in, we celebrated with a bottle of the best—Dom Pérignon!

For the last two and half years, I had focussed on getting well. Where to from here on? Now, I need to sort out a maintenance schedule. I know I need to remain on my 'diet' for the rest of my life. However, it is a small price to pay for good health. My sister has returned home once again, my husband has gone back to work (now in Darwin) to continue financial support, and once again, I will be home alone with my poodles. I intend to remain healthy and to live a long life.

Take-Home Messages

1. Consider seeing a psychologist for support. They can also help to uncover unhealthy or unhelpful beliefs. This is important as beliefs are related to emotions, and emotions are important to our immune system and healing response.
2. If seeing a psychologist is not an option, O. Carl Simonton in his book *The Healing Journey* offers some advice about evaluating beliefs in Chapter 4.
3. Dr O. Carl Simonton also offers us three central beliefs about cancer. These are as follows:

    a. The body has a natural ability to heal itself and overcome cancer. White blood cells routinely attack and destroy weak and confused cancer cells.
    b. Medical treatment will help to heal your body.
    c. Cancer is our feedback that something needs to change. For example, you may need to do more of the things you enjoy and less of the things that cause you pain.

4. Dr O. Carl Simonton also offers, in his book, several guided meditations, including one which uses meditation to decrease the fear of death. He says that we should address this when we feel strong enough, and that the purpose of exploring death is to decrease our fear and, in doing so, increase our energy for living today. He suggests that we examine our beliefs about death and dying and proposes some alternate healthy beliefs such as: we can influence our dying in much the same way as we influence our lives; death is a brief transition between physical life as we know it and an existence that comes after it; and after death, our soul continues on in another existence. He also says, 'The impact of counselling on the course of cancer is solidly documented. Three randomised, match-controlled studies now prove that counselling doubles the expected survival time and improves the quality of life. With counselling, we see increased numbers of long-term survivors and, the "side effects" of counselling are desirable. But there's a resistance to embrace new concepts. That's the problem' (in *Cancer Breakthrough USA—A guide to Outstanding Alternative Clinics* by Frank Cousineau with Andrew Scholberg, Online Publishing and Marketing LLC, 2009).

Once a cancer patient, always a cancer patient. Two such women with Stage IV breast cancer who went into total remission felt that they had beat the disease and jumped off the diet wagon a few years later. Shortly afterwards, their cancers returned with a vengeance.

(Robert Jay Rowen in *Defeat Cancer* by Connie Strasheim, Biomed Publishing Group, 2011)

PART 2
HOW I DID IT

I am aware that there are a lot of strategies mentioned here and further that some people may be overwhelmed by them. I chose to do as many strategies as I could, and I am lucky that the combination worked. It appears that none of them conflicted. As mentioned above, I started on Bill Henderson's protocol, and I did that for twelve months before starting on the Budwig distance programme. Many of these are able to be done at the same time as either Henderson or Budwig. If you choose to do the Budwig distance programme, check with their oncology naturopath before you add anything.

The only strategy I did as a stand-alone was the bicarb-molasses protocol. When I did this for five days, the only supplements I took were selenium, vitamin C, potassium, magnesium, and iodine. On these days, I also drank the AIM products and the Budwig smoothie.

These are the strategies that I utilised:

1. *Protocols*

    a. Bill Henderson, including Beta Glucan 1.3.6, Heart Plus, Vitamin C and Green Tea
    b. Budwig distance programme—Bloodroot, Honokiol, Canelim, Cellect, and others
    c. Bicarb and blackstrap molasses

2. Lifestyle

    a. Sunbathing, vitamin D_3, earthing
    b. Coffee enemas and colonic irrigation
    c. Deep breathing
    d. Dry-skin brushing
    e. Exercise
    f. PEMF
    g. Penne and Poppy, my poodles

3. Supplements

    a. MSM
    b. Iodine
    c. Avemar
    d. Transfer Factor Plus
    e. Melatonin
    f. Magnesium
    g. Probiotics
    h. Artemisinin
    i. Low-dose naltrexone
    j. Fucoidan
    k. Zyflamend
    l. Others, including strontium, vitamin K_2, potassium, Lypo-Spheric Vitamin C, and low-dose lithium

4. Diet

    a. Alkalising
    b. AIM products, Budwig smoothie, and general diet

5. Psychological

    a. *The Journey* and its processes
    b. Meditation
    c. Inspirational stories

Protocols

a) Bill Henderson, including Beta Glucan 1.3.6, Heart Plus, Vitamin C and Green Tea

Transfer Point's Beta Glucan is recommended by Bill Henderson in his e-book *Cancer Free—Your Guide to Gentle, Non-Toxic Healing*. I did the Henderson protocol for about twelve months, and in hindsight, it probably worked during that time. After I had been on the protocol for nearly six months, I had a CT scan which suggested 'increased activity' of my metastases. Although my oncologist suggested that this indicated a worsening of my condition, I refused to believe it, as I felt better, not worse. She offered chemotherapy, but I declined. I think, in hindsight, that my mets were lysing, not getting worse, and this would show as 'increased activity' too.

Bill advocates a number of supplements, and I suspect his protocol does work. He suggests removing root canals, I didn't. He also recommends a vegetarian diet, which I only did for a couple of weeks before starting again to eat organic meat a few times a week. I started to eat meat as my haemoglobin was low. Bill's protocol may well be a good starting point for someone with a non-aggressive cancer. Some of the supplements are not available in Australia and have to be ordered online from the USA. However, some of these companies do not ship to Australia, so you either have to have them sent to a friend in the USA or set up your own mailbox there, and a link to a website which will enable this is given below.

I took Transfer Point's Beta Glucan, an immune modulator, recommended by Bill, on and off. I also took two other supplements recommended by him—Heart Plus and Green Tea, both recommended by Dr Matthias Rath. I got my Heart Plus from ourhealthcoop.com, and the link is given below. Bill provides information about where to get all of his supplements in his book. The booklocker site given below gives a basic outline of his protocol.

Useful websites include the following:

1. http://www.beating-cancer-gently.com/
2. http://www.myus.com/en/landing/?aid=1000721&gclid=CI_H4dXLkLECFaRMpgodY3JCgQ
3. http://www.transferpoint.com/Articles.asp?ID=188
4. http://www.bestbetaglucan.com/
5. http://store.ourhealthcoop.com/category-s/32.htm
6. http://booklocker.com/books/5191.html
7. http://www4.dr-rath-foundation.org/THE_FOUNDATION/scientific_publications.html
8. http://www.cancertutor.com/Cancer/Rath.html

b) Budwig distance programme—Bloodroot, Honokiol, Canelim, Cellect, and others

I started on the Budwig distance programme in July 2011. A fee is paid, and this depends on how many months you intend to stay on the programme. Send an email, and they send back a questionnaire. When that is returned, money is transferred, and the products are sent out. Their oncology naturopath is available for support via email while on the programme. I was on the programme for twelve months. Over the twelve-month period, they used a number of supplements, including Bloodroot, Honokiol, Canelim, and, more recently, Cellect. This protocol is well worth doing as it takes all the hard work out of research. However, it didn't stop me from reading, and while I was on the protocol, I found other supplements such as iodine to take as well. Iodine is now included in their protocol.

Budwig combined with Cellect is described at Cancertutor.com as given below:

'This cancer treatment is one of the crown jewels of alternative medicine! It is the strongest and fastest-acting alternative cancer treatment which does not have any restrictions placed on its use. It does not cause any inflammation or swelling. It frequently shrinks tumours and reduces pain within a couple of weeks. It can be used by any *advanced cancer patient* dealing with any type of cancer.'

Cancertutor.com suggests it is a stage IV treatment.

Useful websites include the following:

1. http://www.budwigcenter.com/
2. http://www.budwigcenter.com/contacts.php
3. http://cancertutor.com/Cancer02/Cellect_Budwig.html

c) Bicarb—blackstrap molasses protocol

I came across this protocol on the Internet. Vernon Johnson claims to have overcome prostate cancer with bone metastases using this protocol. His website is listed below. I contacted him via his website, and he assured me that he is still well and also that one other man has done this successfully. Before undertaking this, it would be wise to speak with your doctor as it may well be contraindicated. I would not do this if I had kidney problems, for example, without consulting with my doctor.

I did this protocol several times and found it scary to do at first as I didn't have support initially. What I found was that I could manage to do this for five days every other month. I took one teaspoon of bicarb with one teaspoon of blackstrap molasses in a glass of water, four times per day for five days. I took this one hour before breakfast, then two hours after breakfast, and one hour before lunch. I then took it two hours after lunch and at least one hour before dinner. Then again, two hours after dinner before bed. I found that this protocol coupled with my barley grass three times per day got my pH up to over 8.0 for the five days. When I initially did it, I found that it reduced my bone pain. When I was on the Zometa IV, I found that my metastases would sometimes burn.

Mark Sircus is available for skype consultations to oversee this protocol, and I did have one with him which was helpful.

Useful websites include the following:

1. http://www.naturalnews.com/035876_baking_soda_cancer_fungus.html
2. http://digitaljournal.com/article/323645
3. http://www.youtube.com/watch?v=Yl8Y8I_TsjI
4. http://imva.info/
5. http://imva.info/index.php/about/consultation/

Lifestyle

a) Sunbathing, vitamin D_3, earthing

I spent time in the sun before 10 a.m. most days. I live in the tropics, so sunbathing after this time is probably not a good idea. I found conflicting information on this, and some sites suggested sunbathing in the middle of the day. As I have fair skin, I didn't want to do this. I stayed in the sun long enough to get a pink tinge on the inside of my arms. I didn't use sunblock, and after the sun exposure, I did not use soap.

While I was sunbathing, I was sitting on a chair in the garden with my bare feet on the ground (earthing). Surprisingly, there appears to be some interest in researching earthing.

Before supplementing with vitamin D_3, ask your GP to check your blood levels.

Useful websites include the following:

1. http://www.cancer.gov/cancertopics/factsheet/prevention/vitamin-D
2. http://www.earthinginstitute.net/
3. http://www.hindawi.com/journals/jeph/2012/291541/
4. http://www.naturalnews.com/009415.html

b) Coffee enemas and colonic irrigation

I started coffee enemas in July 2011 when I commenced the Budwig distance programme. They are recommended by Gerson therapists, and they were recommended by the Budwig programme at that time. They are not sanctioned by mainstream medicine, and as far as I know, there is no evidence base for them. However, I chose to do them. They are done to support the liver and to assist with detoxification. In addition, I read that coffee enemas stimulate tumour necrosis factor, a substance that kills cancer. I found they also help with pain. I did them every day for six months, then three times a week for three months, twice a week for three months, and then once a week. I think they were helpful.

It is time I think that mainstream medicine started to investigate, research, and teach oncologists about alternative and complementary therapies, instead of coming up with articles like this, which I don't think is helpful. I think that instead of criticising these strategies, it would be way more useful to research, given that many people these days are looking outside the medical paradigm for treatment.

http://theconversation.edu.au/coffee-enemas-dont-cure-cancer-reviewing-the-remarkable-claims-of-ian-gawler-5242

My guess is that many people have done as Ian Gawler did and cured their cancers with diet and enemas, despite the fact that in my experience, some oncologists and doctors are just not interested. In my own case, I think that had I done all that my doctors had suggested, including chemo, I would be dead by now, especially given my low neutrophils and white cell count. Of course, there is no way of knowing if this is in fact the case, as I chose not to have chemo. In my opinion, diet and/or supplements can work, and I believe that integrating the two, medicine and complementary therapies, is the way to go. It is also possible, of course, that chemo may work for some people, and for certain cancers, it may well be more efficacious than others.

To make the coffee for the enema, put one litre of filtered, pure water in a saucepan, and add three dessertspoons of organic, ground coffee. Bring to the boil and then simmer with the lid on for twenty minutes. Strain the coffee, cool and add more pure water to make up a litre.

The Budwig Centre recommended doing water enemas first, and I think this does help to hold the coffee. I did two water enemas, first, using one litre of pure water or about 500 ml each time. Then I did the coffee enema. Once the coffee is inside, lie on your right side and hold it for about fifteen to twenty minutes.

I also started a programme of ten colonic irrigations after reading in the cancer e-books that some clinics recommend them for their cancer patients. As far as I am aware, this practice is not evidence based. Alternative sites recommend them, mainstream medicine sites do not. I read that colonics get rid of rubbish in the colon and helps the immune system. Personally, I think these were beneficial too.

Useful websites include the following:

1. http://www.youtube.com/watch?v=BFBkEkYcvKM
2. http://www.cancer-treatment-tips.com/coffee-enema.html
3. http://www.altmd.com/Articles/Colon-Hydrotherapy-for-Cancer
4. http://www.cancer.org/Treatment/TreatmentsandSide Effects/ComplementaryandAlternativeMedicine/ManualHealingandPhysicalTouch/colon-therapy

c) Deep breathing

While I was doing the coffee enemas, I usually did some deep breathing. This was done because I read that it helps oxygenate the body and it can accelerate the elimination of toxins. Is this evidence based? I don't know. I do know that athlete's blood has more oxygen than ordinary people's, and it may well be that this is because of exercise. Apparently, only one in seven athletes will develop cancer as opposed to ordinary people—one in two men or one in three women. Budwig suggest a specific type of breathing, and their link is given below.

Useful websites include the following:

1. http://www.youtube.com/watch?v=wYvMpXCu3mo
2. http://www.adelaide.edu.au/news/news640.html
3. http://www.eurekalert.org/pub_releases/2012-05/uog-lol050312.php

4. http://www.sciencedaily.com/releases/2012/05/120503194219.htm
5. http://www.budwigcenter.com/cancer-breathing-exercises.php

d) Dry-skin brushing

I read that some cancer clinics encourage their patients to do this. It is reported to have several benefits. It helps with elimination of toxins, cleans the pores, exfoliates the skin, keeps skin soft and toned, aids blood circulation, and assists in the optimum functioning of the lymphatic system. I did these after the coffee enemas. Is this evidence based? I don't know, but I figured it wasn't going to do any harm and the very least it could do would be to help smoothen my skin.

Useful websites include the following:

1. http://www.livestrong.com/article/172135-how-to-correctly-dry-brush-your-body/
2. http://www.all-natural-cancer-cures.com/dry-skin-brushing.html

e) Exercise

Regular exercise has a number of benefits. It boosts the immune system and reduces inflammation. It can help boost lymphatic circulation, and it can help reduce stress—all excellent for those with cancer. Exercise can also help prevent cancer from recurring. I walked for about half an hour most days with my poodles.

Discuss exercise with your doctors before embarking on an exercise programme. You will need to recognise your limitations and design your exercise programme to suit yourself.

Useful websites include the following:

1. https://www.caring4cancer.com/go/cancer/wellbeing/physical-wellbeing/exercising-with-cancer-tips-and-more.htm
2. http://www.webmd.com/cancer/features/exercise-cancer-patients

f) Pulse-emitted magnetic field therapy (PEMF)

For those with bone metastases, I can't recommend this highly enough. I used my MRS 2000 which I bought online from pemf.net, every day for three months, three times a day, and then twice a day for six months. I did the whole body mat on 50 per cent in the morning, 25 per cent in the middle of the day, and then 25 per cent later in the afternoon. I found I couldn't go higher than 50 per cent as it kept me awake at night. After three months of using the whole body mat, I then started treating my bone metastases for eight minutes each, twice per day, and I did this for six months. I then reduced my treatment time to once per day.

One of the first uses for PEMF technology was to promote the healing of non-union fractures. Other uses followed with some success. It has been approved by the Federal Drug Administration for bone density and pain management. I found that it did improve my bone density, and it also helped with pain, mood, and, initially, sleep. I also found that it improved my disc protrusion which I have in my lower back. After treating this area for six months daily, I was able to dig again in the garden, something I had not been able to do for years, without experiencing debilitating pain.

With regards to cancer, Cameron et al 2006 conducted experiments with tumour-bearing mice. They found that a standard course of ionising radiation as well as PEMF therapy were both shown to inhibit tumour growth, angiogenesis, and metastasis. In another study, Japanese researchers concluded that PEMF therapy stimulated an immune response which could account for the anti-tumour effect.

Useful websites include the following:

1. http://www.electro-magnetic-therapy.com/pemf-explained/scientific-studies.html
2. http://www.pemf.com/
3. http://pemf.hubpages.com/hub/PEMF-Machines—7-Tips-You-Need-to-Know-Before-Buying

g) Penne and Poppy, my mini poodles

It is well known that owning a pet can benefit your health. Playing with pets can elevate the good hormones, such as serotonin and dopamine. It can also alleviate anxiety and lower blood pressure. Studies of HIV patients with pets suggest that they suffer less depression. Further, heart attack patients with pets survive longer than those without pets. I have no doubt that snuggling with my poodles every day provided me with lots of health benefits, and I strongly recommend pet ownership to anyone dealing with illness.

Useful websites include the following:

1. http://www.webmd.com/hypertension-high-blood-pressure/features/health-benefits-of-pets
2. http://newsinhealth.nih.gov/2009/February/feature1.htm

Supplements

a) MSM (methylsulfonylmethane)

I first became aware of MSM when I read Jerry Nall's story on the Internet. It was one of the products that he used to overcome his prostate cancer with bone mets. MSM is a naturally occurring sulphur compound which reportedly has many uses. It is said to be particularly useful for cancer patients to help reduce inflammation and to assist with pain management. I gradually increased my intake of MSM until I reached a teaspoon of organic MSM twice daily with breakfast and lunch. Do not take MSM after lunch as I read that it can interfere with sleep.

Useful websites include the following:

1. http://www.alkalizeforhealth.net/cancerpain.htm
2. http://www.mismo.com.au/
3. http://www.nwhealthsolutions.com/cancer.htm
4. http://falconblanco.com/health/msm/faq.html

b) Iodine

I read Mark Sircus's e-books on cancer and started to read about iodine. This led to David Brownstein, and I read his book *Iodine: Why You Need It and Why You Can't Live Without It*. Despite the inevitable claims of 'quackery' from several sources, I was quite excited when I read this. Like so many other perimenopausal women, I have fibrocystic breasts, a precursor to breast cancer. I read that iodine supplementation can improve this condition, and to my surprise, it did. When I went off the iodine, the condition came back as evidenced by ultrasounds.

Brownstein also claims that iodine downregulates oestrogen receptors in the breast and upregulates the BRCA genes. He also says that at 50 mg daily, iodine induces apoptosis in cancer cells.

Before taking iodine, I think it is a good idea to be tested, and there are a couple of laboratories in the USA which offer the iodine-loading test. If you have breast cancer, it would also be a good idea to have the bromide test done at the same time. The link to the lab is given below.

When taking iodine, I found it best to build up slowly, and I started on Lugol's iodine half strength. Start with a couple of drops and build up over a couple of months to 50 mg or more. Companion nutrients, vitamin C, magnesium, and selenium as well as ½ teaspoon Himalayan rock salt should be taken as well. I took the cofactors, vitamin B_2 (riboflavin) and B_3 (niacin) for a while but didn't like the niacin flush, so I stopped.

Stephanie Buist, a Canadian naturopath and a thyroid cancer survivor, is available for skype consultation to assist with this. She is the moderator of an Iodine Facebook site and Yahoo! Group, and her website is listed below. I tried to find doctors here who knew about iodine supplementation and couldn't find one. Those with thyroid conditions should consult their doctors before starting iodine supplementation.

Breastcancerchoices.org (link below) provides a useful summary and instructions.

Note that fluoride takes up iodine receptors, so drinking pure water is recommended.

Selenium comes in different forms, and I took 200 mcg Se-methyl L-selenocysteine daily, from the Life Extension Foundation (link given below). The NaturalNews website, given below, provides a nice summary of selenium.

I bought some of my Lugol's online from an Australian website, but I became frustrated because some of the liquid seemed stronger than others, and I wasn't absolutely sure what dose I was getting, so I found a website in Australia which sold Iodoral.

Mark Sircus recommends nascent iodine; however, this is quite expensive, and once again, I found a website which sells it in Australia but found that it was unreliable and did not know exactly what strength it was. La Diosa, where I bought my Iodoral, (link 9 given below) also sells magnesium products. David Brownstein recommends either Iodoral or Lugol's. Lugol's is handy for painting.

I found that painting the inside of my wrists whenever I got a sore throat stopped the progression of colds. Mark Sircus also recommends painting the breasts, and this can be done too. This caused some dryness and irritation, so I also massaged on hemp seed oil or coconut oil at night.

Useful websites include the following:

1. http://drdavidbrownstein.blogspot.com.au/
2. http://health.groups.yahoo.com/group/iodine/
3. https://www.facebook.com/iodineskyband#!/groups/iodine4health/
4. http://breastcancerchoices.org/iodine.html
5. http://www.naturalnews.com/016446.html
6. http://www.lef.org/Vitamins-Supplements/Item00567/Se-Methyl-L-Selenocysteine-SeMC.html
7. http://cancerpreventionresearch.aacrjournals.org/content/2/7/683.short
8. http://www.strideintohealth.com/Lugols-Solution.html
9. http://www.bestofthebest.net.au/supplement_sydney_australia/index.html

10. http://www.hakalalabs.com/ (Iodine loading test)
11. http://steppingstonesliving.com/resources/iodine/

c) Avemar

I took Avemar, a fermented wheatgerm product, for about six months initially. It is reasonably expensive, but the research behind it is impressive. Apparently, it is routinely prescribed for cancer patients in Hungary, where it was developed. I obtained mine from a health professional and could not find it anywhere else. It needs to be refrigerated, so look for it in health-food shop fridges.

According to betterhealthinternational.com, it works in the following manner:

- Avemar regulates and modulates the immune system so that all white blood cells do exactly what they are supposed to do at precisely the right time.
- Avemar exposes harmful cells that are hiding from the immune system so that they can be destroyed by your body's natural killer (NK) cells.
- Avemar helps to starve harmful cells by depriving them of the massive amounts of glucose they need to survive.

I found one Australian website which offers it for sale, and it is listed below.

Useful websites include the following:

1. http://www.avemarcancertreatment.com/?gclid=CJbL08LKjrECFUskpQodun1okA
2. http://www.avemar.com.au/orders.ews

Transfer Factor Plus

This was taken as an immune system stimulant. Their website says . . .

'Also features an advanced and proprietary blend of transfer factors, plus other natural components from cow colostrum. However, 4Life Transfer Factor Plus contains Cordyvant, our advanced and proprietary blend of extra-helpful ingredients such as shiitake mushrooms, maitake mushrooms, cordyceps, and beta-glucan.'

I noticed that this appeared on the Budwig schedule, but it was not provided by them. There are some impressive testimonials about this product, and the link is given below.

Useful websites include the following:

1. http://www.4tf.com/
2. http://www.youtube.com/watch?v=1-eMQTGnCdw
3. http://projects.alexmed.edu.eg/journal/index.php/bulletin/article/view/287
4. http://cancer-treatment-registry.org/make-cancer-treatment.php?treatment_id=78
5. http://transferfactortestimonies.blogspot.com.au/2007/10/cancer-hodgkins-product-testimonials.htm

d) Melatonin

Women with breast cancer have been found to have lower levels of melatonin. Melatonin is a hormone produced in the brain by the pineal gland. Production is triggered by darkness and stopped by light. It is reported to reduce circulating oestrogen levels, inhibit syntheses of oestrogen, and increase immune function. I also took it as it stimulates the production of interleukin-4 in bone marrow T-lymphocytes. Check with your doctor or oncology pharmacist before taking melatonin. I have taken anywhere from 5 to 25 mg. Breastcancerchoices.org suggests that we can take up to 50 mg indefinitely.

Useful websites include the following:

1. http://www.mskcc.org/cancer-care/herb/melatonin
2. http://www.umm.edu/altmed/articles/melatonin-000315.htm
3. http://www.naturalmedicinejournal.com/article_content.asp?article=108
4. http://www.breastcancerchoices.org/melatonin.html

e) Magnesium

I read about magnesium in Mark Sircus's books initially. Magnesium is essential for cellular survival and the removal of toxins and acid residues. It is depleted by alcohol consumption, some pharmaceuticals, radiation, and chemotherapy. Magnesium is found in leafy greens, nuts, and legumes.

Some research has been done in the field of magnesium and cancer. For example, researchers from the School of Public Health at the University of Minnesota suggested that diets rich in magnesium reduce the risk of colon cancer. Furthermore, a Swedish study reported that women with the highest magnesium intake had a 40 per cent lower risk of developing cancer than those with a lower intake.

Mark recommends the use of transdermal as well as oral magnesium chloride. He suggests that it could take three to four months for a cancer patient to achieve saturation at the cellular level. Before adding magnesium to your regime, it would be wise to check with your doctor or oncology pharmacist as there may well be contraindications, for example, those with kidney problems.

Useful websites include the following:

1. http://www.naturalnews.com/023279_magnesium_cancer_calcium.html#ixzz20jsWly78
2. http://www.canceractive.com/cancer-active-page-link.aspx?n=522
3. http://www.winningcancer.com/txt/fundamental-methodology/

f) Probiotics

According to breastcancerconqueror.com, probiotics are necessary for immune functioning and absorption of nutrients and work on several levels:

1. They fight off unhealthy organisms and reduce the risk of infection.
2. They regulate Immune responses.
3. They help fight inflammatory responses and reduce your risk of cancer.
4. They support the healthy function of elimination from the colon.
5. They even have an effect on allergies and obesity.

I took one most days and continue to do so.

Useful websites include the following:

1. http://breastcancerconqueror.com/probiotics-and-cancer/
2. http://www.ncbi.nlm.nih.gov/pubmed/17922945

g) Artemisinin

Artemisinin has been used to treat malaria and parasite infestations. It reacts with a high concentration of iron, and this reaction creates free radicals that attack cell membranes, breaking them apart and killing them. Cancer cells have many more iron-attracting receptors than do healthy cells. As artemisinin binds to iron, the theory is that it also binds to cancer cells. If you decide to take artemisinin, you will need to do your homework.

I took it for ten days at a time, five tablets in the morning and five at night (dose based on mg/kg). I took this many tablets based on my weight at the time. I also took it with flaxseed oil and cottage cheese as it needs oil to be absorbed. I also supplemented with iron in between a couple of times to boost my iron levels. This is not a stand-alone therapy, and you will need to discuss this therapy with your doctor. Blood tests may be necessary, and it may be contraindicated.

Useful websites include the following:

1. http://www.mnwelldir.org/docs/cancer1/altthrpy.htm#Artemisinin
2. http://artemisinin.pbworks.com/w/page/13759315/FrontPage
3. http://www.naturalnews.com/033182_artemisinin_cancer.html
4. http://www.mwt.net/~drbrewer/FreeCanArtimisUpDate.htm

h) Low-dose naltrexone

I found out about this late in 2011 and had to educate my doctors as it is unheard of here.

Dr Bernard Bihari pioneered work with low-dose naltrexone (LDN) in 1986. He discovered that it could help protect people with HIV by enhancing their response to the infection. In the 1990s, he further found that naltrexone in low doses could also help cancer patients and those with autoimmune diseases. Naltrexone had been approved by the FDA in 1984 for the purpose of helping those with heroin or opium addictions, by blocking the effect of those drugs. By blocking opiod receptors, naltrexone also blocks the reception of opioid hormones that our brain and adrenal glands produce—beta endorphin and metenkephalin. Many body tissues have receptors for these, including nearly every cell of our immune system.

Research has demonstrated inhibition of a number of different human tumours in laboratory studies by using endorphins and LDN. LDN (4.5 mg) taken between 9 p.m. and 10 p.m. every day results in increased endorphin and enkephalin levels between 2 a.m. and 4 a.m., and this works directly on tumour's opiod receptors. Furthermore, it is believed that they act to increase natural killer cell activity, and other healthy immune defences against cancer.

I mixed my own LDN. My pharmacist gave me a brown 110 ml bottle filled with distilled water, and I crushed two 50-mg tablets into this. When starting to take LDN, take 1.5 mg per night for a month and build up by 1 mg every month until you get to the therapeutic dose 4.5 mg. This minimises side effects. If you consider LDN, please visit the second website given below and think about participating in a clinical trial if you meet the criteria. There is a Yahoo! group, and the link for this is given below.

Useful websites include the following:

1. http://www.lowdosenaltrexone.org/
2. http://www.transparencyls.com/
3. http://csn.cancer.org/node/221154

4. http://www.mbschachter.com/protocol_for_low.htm
5. http://health.groups.yahoo.com/group/lowdosenaltrexone/

i) Fucoidan

I started on this in early 2012 when I read about it on cancertutor.com. In 1996, researchers in Japan discovered that U-fucoidan, found in brown seaweed Laminaria japonica, induces apoptosis in cancer cells.

I took four a day for six months and then two per day. I bought mine from posiedonsharvest.com and the link is given below.

Useful websites include the following:

1. http://www.ncbi.nlm.nih.gov/sites/entrez?term=fucoidan%20cancer%C2%A0%C2%A0
2. http://www.raysahelian.com/fucoidan.html
3. http://www.cancertutor.com/Cancer03/LimuJuice.html
   http://www.poseidonsharvest.com/u-fn/
4. http://www.ncbi.nlm.nih.gov/pubmed?term=apoptosis%20fucoidan

j) Zyflamend

My erythrocyte sedimentation rate (ESR) level, a non-specific measure of inflammation, was quite high, and apparently, this is common with metastatic breast cancer. Dr Jenkins, the oncology naturopath at the Budwig Cancer Centre, recommended Zyflamend. My ESR levels came down significantly within six months. This is a herbal anti-inflammatory drug, and although it is herbal, it is still powerful. I took three a day initially, and my platelets were adversely affected, so I cut back to two per day which is the recommended dose. As far as I am aware, this product is not available in Australia and has to be shipped from the USA. I got mine from New Chapter, and their link is given below. Since I ordered mine initially, it seems they have developed new products which target specific areas, such as breast health. Before ordering this, please check with your doctor or treating health practitioner to ensure there aren't any contraindications.

Useful websites include the following:

1. http://www.newchapter.com/zyflamend/zyflamend-whole-body
2. http://www.newchapter.com/zyflamend
3. http://jco.ascopubs.org/content/27/21/3418.full

k) Others including strontium, vitamin K_2, potassium, Lypo-Spheric Vitamin C, low-dose lithium

Stable strontium, as opposed to strontium-90, a radioactive compound, appears to be effective for the treatment of osteoporosis and other bone-related diseases. It has been safely used for more than one hundred years. It should be taken on an empty stomach, and it should not be taken with calcium or calcium-containing supplements. I got mine from Swanson's Vitamins online, and their link is given below.

Vitamin K_2 works to help maintain healthy bone mass and growth. One of the best food sources is a Japanese fermented food called Natto. Its benefits are enhanced when combined with vitamin D_3. Vitamin D_3 encourages calcium uptake to promote strong, healthy bones.

I took potassium when I was doing the bicarb-molasses protocol. I did this because it was recommended by Vernon in his site.

According to LivOn Laboratories, Lypo-Spheric Vitamin C 'is encapsulated in liposomes and as a result is able to cross the normal barriers to absorption into the cells'. Their link is given below. I got mine from John Appleton, and his link is given below.

I took low-dose lithium orotate after reading about it in the link (8) given below. Very low amounts of lithium can influence brain function for the better as well as possibly aid a low white cell count (see link 10 below).

Useful websites include the following:

1. http://www.worldhealth.net/news/strontium_breakthrough_against_osteoporo/
2. http://www.nps.org.au/consumers/publications/medicine_update/issues/strontium_ranelate
3. http://www.swansonvitamins.com/DB116/ItemDetail
4. http://products.mercola.com/vitamin-k/
5. http://www.iherb.com/Thorne-Research-Vitamin-K2-1-fl-oz-30-ml/21592?at=0
6. http://phkillscancer.com/vitamins_minerals_herbs
7. http://www.livonlabs.com/
8. http://www.johnappleton.co.nz/products/Lypo%252dSpheric-Vitamin-C.html
9. http://tahomaclinicblog.com/lithium-the-misunderstood-mineral-part-1/
10. http://tahomaclinicblog.com/lithium-the-misunderstood-mineral-part-2/
11. http://www.globalhealingcenter.com/natural-health/lithium-orotate/

Diet

a) Alkalising

I read that cancer cells survive in a low-oxygen state. When our cells and tissues are acidic (below a pH of 6.5-7.0), they lose their ability to exchange oxygen, but cancer cells thrive. When cells and tissues are alkaline (above pH of 7.0), cancer cells do not thrive because of the high amount of oxygen present. I also read that cancer will not survive in a pH of 8.0 and above.

I measured my saliva and urine pH using sticks and strips and found this confusing. There is a difference between sticks and strips, and I also found a difference between my saliva and urine pH. I also read that the bigger the difference, the more problems there are with digestion. How true is this? I don't know. I eventually stuck with testing my urine pH, and tested the second one of the day with strips, not sticks. The pH testing kits can be obtained generally from health-food shops. They can also be bought online.

I found I could not alkalise without using alkalising drops for my drinking water. There are also websites which suggest which foods are alkaline and which are acid forming.

To raise my pH to 8.0 and above, I did Vernon Johnson's bicarb-molasses protocol once a month every other month for five days. I took one teaspoon of bicarb and one teaspoon of molasses in a glass of water when I got up in the morning. I then waited one hour before eating. I then drank another glass at least two hours later and one hour before eating lunch. Two hours after lunch and at least one hour before eating dinner, I drank another glass. Then two hours after dinner, I drank my last glass for the day. This, along with my barley grass before meals, raised my pH to 8.0 and above. I found I couldn't stomach more than four teaspoons for five days. I would not do this for longer than five days.

The molasses is supposed to take the bicarb up to the tumours. Given the PET/CT scans use a sugar solution, I think this is reasonable to assume that this is in fact the case.

Most mornings I had half teaspoon of Alkala N in a glass of water with some lemon juice, and this also helped to keep me in the 7.0 to 7.5 pH range. It is available online at quantamwellness.com.au, and their link is given below.

Useful websites include the following:

1. http://www.alternative-cancer-care.com/pH_Cancer_Alkaline.html—this is typical of many alkalising and cancer websites
2. http://www.alkaway.com.au
3. http://www.acidalkalinediet.com/Alkaline-Foods-Chart.htm
4. http://phkillscancer.com/
5. http://www.naturalhealth365.com/cancer/baking-soda.html
6. http://www.quantumwellness.com.au/

b) AIM products, Budwig smoothie, and general diet

The diet I stuck with was mostly gluten free, dairy free (except for quark in the Budwig smoothie), sugar free, alcohol free, caffeine free, and mainly vegetarian. I did not eat processed foods and made my own gluten-free sweets using stevia. I found that most recipes can be adjusted. Low carb is the best. When I did eat meat, I ate organic beef or chicken, and I had the occasional Tasmanian salmon.

I bought BarleyLife, Just Carrots and RediBeets as well as Herbal Fibreblend and Pro Peas from AIM. I drank barley grass three times a day about half hour before meals. Every day for lunch, I had a barley grass, carrot and beetroot juice, and the Budwig smoothie. To make the smoothie: Blend with a stick blender one and half tablespoons flaxseed oil (always buy refrigerated oil, not from the supermarket shelf) and three tablespoons quark until all the oil is absorbed. Grind one tablespoon fresh flaxseed, six apricot kernels, and one tablespoon chia seeds, then add to the oil and quark. I then added berries, banana, and almond milk to make the smoothie. The link to instructions to the smoothie is given below.

Breakfast was mostly a gluten-free cereal with almond milk or occasional muesli with oat milk. I usually added some Pro Peas to my cereal to increase protein and enzymes.

Useful websites include the following:

1. http://www.ivanhoe.com/channels/p_channelstory.cfm?storyid=28587
2. http://www.sciencedaily.com/releases/2011/06/110614115037.htm
3. http://www.cancerproject.org/ask/dairy.php
4. http://www.naturalnews.com/030403_cancer_cure.html
5. http://www.naturalnews.com/028145_gluten_intolerance_cancer.html
6. http://www.livestrong.com/article/468494-is-gluten-bad-for-people-with-cancer/
7. http://breastcancer.about.com/od/cancerfightingfoods/a/cancer_sugar_myth.htm
8. http://www.youtube.com/watch?v=RSoddptWL0s
9. http://www.all-natural-cancer-cures.com/the-china-study.html

10. http://www.budwigcenter.com/anti-cancer-diet.php
11. http://www.naturalnews.com/036455_gluten_sensitivity_flour.html

Psychological

a) The Journey and its processes

A friend of my cousin's lent me this book. Brandon Bays, the author, wrote the book after she was diagnosed with a mass in her stomach. She started on a programme of raw food, supplements, and emotional healing, and about two months later, she was healthy—no more mass.

In her book *The Journey*, she describes a process for getting to the 'source' and for resolving long-standing issues. I did the processes by myself, and each one takes about two hours. They are very cathartic, and I am grateful that my husband was there for comfort at the end of each session. These processes are highly recommended.

I have no doubt that the onset of my metastases was stress related, although a direct cause-and-effect relationship has apparently not been proven between stress and cancer. Evidence does suggest, however, that chronic stress weakens a person's immune system, and this in turn may render the body more vulnerable to cancer.

Useful websites include the following:

1. http://www.thejourney.com/
2. http://www.cancer.gov/cancertopics/factsheet/Risk/stress

b) Meditation

In the last twenty years, meditation has been studied in clinical trials as a way of reducing stress, and the evidence suggests that it can help reduce anxiety, stress, blood pressure, chronic pain, and insomnia. In one study of ninety cancer patients, those who meditated for seven weeks had reduced stress levels and also fewer episodes of mood disturbance than those who did not meditate. In a study of sixty breast cancer survivors, women who practiced meditation had reduced number and severity of hot flashes and also reported improvements in mood and sleep. Some studies have suggested that more meditation improves the chance of a positive outcome.

Dr O. Carl Simonton in his book *The Healing Journey* describes how to do a series of meditations, and these are well worth doing. They are as follows:

1. Changing beliefs about cancer
2. Developing trust
3. Communicating with your inner wisdom
4. Increasing your trust in yourself through working with pain
5. Increasing your energy for getting well by decreasing the fear of death

Dr Simonton suggests that there are at least three systems in the body that can communicate emotions at the physical level. These include the endocrine system which communicates via hormones, the nervous system which connects to the white blood cells, and also the communication molecules such as neuropeptides and neurotransmitters which not only influence cellular activity but also affect cell division and genetic functioning. He concludes that there is much evidence now to support the fact that the state of mind influences the course of cancer as well as other serious illnesses.

I did meditations twice per day before I got out of bed and before I went to sleep. I focussed on healing images and developed my meditation with the assistance of Dr Simonton's book. I also did the other meditations as outlined by Dr Simonton.

Useful websites include the following:

1. http://www.cancercouncil.com.au/901/get-informed/complementary-treatment/meditation/cancer-council-new-south-wales-meditation-for-people-with-cancer-their-families-and-carers/?pp=901
2. http://www.melbournemeditationcentre.com.au/products/details.php?code=book_eh3&author=1
3. http://www.huffingtonpost.com/joseph-nowinski-phd/cancer-meditation_b_858954.html
4. http://www.meditationexpert.com/health-relaxation/h_meditation_methods_to_help_fight_cancer.htm
5. http://www.simontoncenter.com/
6. http://thehealingjournal.com/node/1447

c) Inspirational stories

Whenever I had a down day, or started to feel some doubt or anxiety, I found looking at inspirational cancer stories uplifting. They inspired me to continue and to reinforce that I could do this. They gave me hope and fuelled my determination.

I had downloaded reports on alternative cancer centres in Europe and the USA, and reading these also inspired me as they had survivor stories in them. These links are given below. I found that reading these also gave me information which I used to help myself. Reading all the information on cancertutor.com also helped me to stay motivated and to believe that I could recover from metastatic breast cancer.

Many of the cancer e books can be found online (link 10 below).

Another very useful resource can be found at link 11 below. The Alternative Cancer Research Institute has published a book called the *Complete Guide to Alternative Cancer Treatments*. If this book is ordered, three additional reports come with it. One of these is called *I Beat Cancer* and contains the testimonials of 1500 survivors who detail which therapies they used to overcome their particular cancers. It also includes links to the therapies. I was quite excited when I found this resource—it is wonderful.

Useful websites include the following:

1. http://radiologytechnicianschools.net/top-50-cancer-survival-inspiration-blogs/
2. http://phkillscancer.com/
3. http://cancertutor.com/index.html
4. http://www.germancancerbreakthrough.com/B/
5. http://www.germancancerbreakthrough.com/B/
6. http://cancerbreakthroughusa.com/
7. http://adios-cancer.com/
8. http://chrisbeatcancer.com/a-matter-of-life-sneak-peak-trailer/
9. https://www.facebook.com/#!/pages/Cure-Cancer-Naturally/360884368785
10. http://www.cancerdefeated.com/About/
11. http://www.alternativecancerresearchinstitute.com/
12. http://www.alternative-cancer-care.com/Lothar_Hirneise.html

Useful Facebook sites include the following:

1. https://www.facebook.com/#!/Alternativehealthsolutions1

2. https://www.facebook.com/pages/Cure-Cancer-Naturally/360884368785
3. https://www.facebook.com/#!/pages/Cancer-Cures-What-They-Dont-Want-You-To-Know/125520664180633
4. https://www.facebook.com/KickCancerCrew?ref=ts
5. https://www.facebook.com/SimontonCenter
6. https://www.facebook.com/Iodine4Health
7. https://www.facebook.com/thesleepdoctor
8. https://www.facebook.com/VitaminAdvisor
9. https://www.facebook.com/pages/There-is-a-cure-for-Cancer-but-it-is-not-FDA-approved-Phoenix-Tears-work/395190597537
10. https://www.facebook.com/pages/NaturalHealth365com/213274862038892?sk=wall

Table 1: **Protein food chart**
(we need about 1 gram per kilo of bodyweight per day)

Food	Portion	Grams of protein (approx.)
Lentils	1 cup	17
Chickpeas	1 cup	15
Kidney beans	1 cup	15
Tofu (firm with nigari)	½ cup	20
Miso	1 tablespoon	2
Flax seeds (whole)	1 tablespoon	1.5
Sesame seeds	1 tablespoon	1.6
Almonds	½ oz	3
Cashew	1 oz	2.5
Peanut paste	1 tablespoon	4
Brown rice	1 cup	5
Millet	1 cup	6
Oats	1 cup	5
Quinoa	1 cup	8
Japanese soba noodles	1 cup	6
Asparagus	½ cup	2
Broccoli	½ cup	3
Green peas	½ cup	4
Mushrooms—oyster raw	½ cup	2.4
Potato with skin baked	1 medium	4
Spinach	½ cup	2.6
Spirulina	1 tablespoon	4

Source: http://www.savvyvegetarian.com/articles/get-enough-protein-veg-diet.php.

Table 2: **Food sources of magnesium** (the current recommended daily intake is 350 mg but there is growing evidence that this is not sufficient)

Food	Portion	Mg (approx.)
Brazil nuts	30 g (approx. 1 oz)	107
Quinoa	¼ cup	89
Almonds	30 g	78
Spinach	½ cup	78
Cashews	30 g	74
Pine nuts	30 g	71
Brown rice	½ cup	42
Tofu (firm with nigari)	½ cup	47
Banana	1	50
Grapes—white	20	6
Orange	1	18
Watermelon	180 g	19
Lentils	50 g	44
Broccoli	45 g	5
Potato with skin on	260 g	62
Spinach	100 gr	59
Millet	50 g	92
Raspberries	75 g	16.5
Chickpeas	50 g	90
Mango	160 g	29
Kidney beans	50 g	101
Carrots—raw	60 g	7

Source: *Dietary Healing*, Kathryn Alexander, 2007; Annexus Pty Ltd.

Table 3: **Non-dairy sources of calcium**
(women aged >50 need 1200 mg daily)

Food	Portion	Ca (approx.)
Banana	1	8
Grapes (white)	20	20
Orange	1	57
Raspberries	75 g	30
Brazil Nuts	40 g	72
Cashews	40 g	15
Almonds	40 g	100
Sunflower Seeds	40 g	52
Chickpeas	50 g	84
Kidney beans	50 g	78
Lentils	50 g	22
Tofu	50 g	257
Avocado	½ cup	11
Broccoli	45 g	34
Carrots raw	60 g	28
Leeks	160 g	97
Peas	80 g	24
Potato with skin	260 g	20
Spinach	100 g	600
Brown rice	50 g	37
Millet	50 g	23
Oats	50 g	60

Source: *Dietary Healing*,
Kathryn Alexander, 2007; Annexus Pty Ltd.

Table 4: **Acid and alkaline food chart**

Healthy alkaline foods	Consume moderately	Acidic food— try to avoid
Asparagus	Apples	Beef
Barley grass	Apricots	Chicken
Broccoli	Bananas	Eggs
Brussel sprouts	Blueberries	Ocean fish
Cabbage	Cantaloupe	Organ meats
Lettuce	Grapes	Pork
Cauliflower	Grapefruit	Veal
Celery	Mandarin	Buttermilk
Chives	Mango	Cream
Cucumber	Orange	Hard cheese
Green beans	Papaya	Homogenised milk
Leeks	Peach	Quark
Peas	Pear	Rye bread
Red cabbage	Pineapple	White biscuit
Garlic	Raspberries	White bread
Spinach	Strawberries	Wholegrain bread
Beetroot	Watermelon	Wholemeal bread
Zucchini	Brown rice	Cashews
Carrot	Wheat	Peanuts
Potatoes	Hazlenuts	Pistachios
Radish	Macadamias	Butter
Turnip	Walnuts	Corn oil
Avocado	Fresh water fish	Margarine
Lemons	Coconut milk	Artificial sweeteners
Limes	Sunflower oil	Chocolate
Tomatoes	Cherries	Fructose
Lentils	Coconut	Honey
Quinoa	Cranberries	Milk sugar
Spelt	Currants	Molasses
Tofu	Dates	White sugar

Almonds		Tomato sauce (Ketchup)
Brazil nuts		Mayonnaise
Flax seeds		Mustard
Sesame seeds		Soy sauce
Sunflower seeds		Vinegar
Flaxseed oil		Beer
Olive oil		Coffee
		Fruit juice
		Tea
		Wine

Source: http://www.balance-ph-diet.com/acid_alkaline_food_chart.html.

MEDICAL REPORTS

JEFFERY, DENICE

KEWARRA BEACH QLD 4879
Birthdate: XXXXXX
Telephone: XXXXXXXXXXX
Your Reference: XX Lab Reference: XXX
Addressee: XXX Referred by: XXXX
Copy to: DR XXXXXXXXX
Name of Test: **MR ARTHROGRAM RIGHT SHOULDER**
Requested: 02/03/2010 Collected: 19/03/2010
Requested tests: Arthrography—Double contrast R side, MRI musc. Skel. R SHOULDER
Laboratory: QUEENSLAND X-RAY REPORTS
Phone enquiries: CAIRNS XXXXXXXXXXX (07) 40467800

MR ARTHROGRAM RIGHT SHOULDER

History: Two year history of right shoulder pain? Cuff tear or labral injury or impingement.

Technique: Under fluoroscopic guidance, sterile technique and local anaesthetic a combination of iodine and Gadolinium contrast was infused into the right shoulder joint via a posterior approach. This was followed by proton density fat suppression axial images, T1 weighted and proton density fat suppression sagittal images and T1 weighted and T2 weighted fat suppression coronal images.

Findings: Abnormal signal with replacement of fatty marrow is seen within the humeral shaft and head and also within the glenoid, acromion and distal clavicle. I note the patient has had previous breast cancer and the appearances are highly suspicious fpr extensive metastatic disease. No definite fracture is identified. The labrum and rotator cuff and biceps tendons are all intact. The glenohumeral ligaments are intact. No significant impingement or bursitis is apparent although minor degenerative changes are seen in the AC joint. No further significant pathology is seen.

Conclusion: Widespread metastatic disease in the bones around the right shoulder but with no obvious fracture. I note a previous bone scan of 23/05/2008 showed no significant abnormality in this region but a repeat bone scan may be of benefit to assess any interval change. No other significant pathology is seen around the shoulder.

Thank you for referring this patient.

Dr XXXXXXXXXXXXXXXXXXXXXX
cc: Dr XXXXXXXXXXXXXXXXXXXXX

This is an official medical report. If you are not the intended recipient please contact our radiology practice immediately and advise us.

QUEENSLAND X-RAY PTY LTD ABN: XXXXXXXXXXXXXX
Cairns XXXXXX, CAIRNS QLD 4870
Telephone: (07) 40467800 Facsimile: (07) 40467820

Wednesday, 24 March 2010
DR XXXXXXXXXXXXXXXXXX
Raintrees Shopping Centre
Manunda Qld 4870

RE: **MRS DENICE JEFFERY** Patient ID: XXXXXXXXXXXXXX
Service Date: 24/03/2010
Dept:
UR No:

BONE SCAN

History: MRI of right shoulder suspicious for mets.

Findings: Since the previous bone scan of 23/05/2008, multiple foci of increased uptake are seen particularly around the right scapula, diffusely within the spine, ribs, pelvis, skull vault and proximal humeri and femora. The appearances are highly suspicious for widespread metastatic deposit. No further significant pathology is seen.

Conclusion: Widespread bony metastases which have developed since the previous bone scan.

Thank you for referring this patient.

Dr: XXXXXXXXXXXXXXXXX

This is an official medical report. If you are not the intended recipient please contact our radiology practice immediately and advise us.

QUEENSLAND X-RAY PTY LTD ABN: XXXXX
Cairns XXXXXX, CAIRNS QLD 4870
Telephone: (07) 40467800 Facsimile: (07) 40467820

Saturday, 27 March 2010
DR: XXXXXXXXXXXXXXXXXXXX

RE: **MRS DENICE JEFFERY** Patient ID: xxx
KEWARRA BEACH Q 4879
Service Date: 27/03/2010
Dept:
UR No:

CT BRAIN, NECK, CHEST, ABDOMEN AND PELVIS

Clinical information: Metastatic breast Ca.

Technique: Post IV contrast axial scans obtained through the brain, chest, abdomen and pelvis.

No previous body Ct available on the system for comparison.

CT BRAIN

Findings: No enhancing mass lesion evident. Ventricles are within normal limits. No intra or extra axial haemorrhage.

CT NECK, CHEST, ABDOMEN AND PELVIS

Findings: No lymphadenopathy in the neck, perihilar or paratracheal regions. There is a 7 mm rounded nodule at the right apex with a much smaller 1 mm nodule in the left upper lobe laterally. These are non-specific but given the clinical history is concerning for metastatic lesions. There are a couple of posterior pleural tags in the upper zones with subpleural lines in the right anterior mid and lower zones. There are a couple of low density lesions in the liver. The largest is in segment 7 measuring approximately 1.3×1.2 cm, density reading would suggest fluid within the lesions but an ultrasound would be useful for further evaluation. Kidneys are contrasting normally. No paraaortic lymphadenopathy. The uterus is quite bulky and inhomogeneous suggesting presence of fibroids. Dominant right ovarian follicle demonstrated. No free fluid. No gross bowel abnormality evident. Quite extensive sclerotic lesions throughout the bone in keeping with diffuse bony metastasis.

This is an official medical report. If you are not the intended recipient, please contact our radiology practice immediately and advise us.

QUEENSLAND X-RAY PTY LTD ABN: XXXXX
Cairns XXXXXX, CAIRNS QLD 4870
Telephone: (07) 40467800 Facsimile: (07) 49467820

Comment: Metastatic bone disease. Two non-specific nodules in the upper lobes bilaterally. Low density lesions in the liver, likely cysts, but ultrasound is suggested for further evaluation.

Thank you for referring this patient.

DR: XXXXXXXXXXXXXXXXX

This is an official medical report. If you are not the intended recipient, please contact our radiology practice immediately and advise us.

QUEENSLAND X-RAY PTY LTD ABN: XXXXX
Cairns XXXXXX, CAIRNS QLD 4870
Telephone: (07) 40467800 Facsimile: (07) 49467820

Monday, 15 November 2010
CAIRNS XXXXXX
CAIRNS QLD 4870

RE: **MRS DENICE JEFFERY** Patient ID:
KEWARRA BEACH QLD 4879
Service Date: 15/11/2010
Dept:
UR No:

BONE SCAN

History: Metastatic breast cancer? Progress

Findings: Since the previous bone scan of 24/03/2010 there is an overall impression of increased activity throughout the spine and pelvis and the multiple metastatic deposits seen on the earlier study in the right scapula, T12 vertebral body and right pubic ramis are more prominent. The appearances are of increased diffuse metastatic disease since the earlier study. No further new pathology is seen.

Conclusion: There has been an increase in size and intensity of the metastatic deposits previously noted and there is diffuse increased activity within the spine and pelvis all consistent with increased metastatic deposits from the earlier study.

Thank you for referring this patient.

DR: XXXXXXXXXXXXXXX
cc: DR XXXXXXXXXXXXXXXXXXXX
DR XXXXXXXXXXXXXXXXXXXXXXXX

This is an official medical report. If you are not the intended recipient, please contact our radiology practice immediately and advise us.

QUEENSLAND X-RAY PTY LTD ABN: XXXXX
XXXXXX Hospital Brisbane, SOUTH BRISBANE QLD 4101
Telephone: (07) 38406200 Facsimile: (07) 38461987

Monday, 18 June 2012
CAIRNS XXXXXX
CAIRNS QLD 4870

RE: **MRS DENICE JEFFERY** Patient ID:
KEWARRA BEACH QLD 4879
Service Date: 18/06/12
Dept:
UR No:
Episode ID:

POSITRON EMISSON TOMOGRAPHY AND CT HEAD, NECK, CHEST, ABDOMEN, PELVIS

Clinical History: Metastatic breast cancer with bone mets. Hormonal therapy. Progress

Technique: 230 MBq of F18-FDG was injected via a left cubital fossa vein. The BSL was 5.4 mmol/-PET images were acquired from the vertex to the mid thighs.

CT images were acquired spirally through the head, neck, chest, abdomen, pelvis and proximal femora following intravenous injection of iodinated contrast.

PET and diagnostic images were fused and reviewed on the workstation.

Findings: Comparison is made with the previous PET CT of 15/12/2010.

Brain: No change since the previous examination. Left maxillary antral polyp unchanged. No pathologic enhancement or abnormal Ct density. No evidence of cranial metastatic disease.

Neck: The previously demonstrated mildly enlarged left cervical node between sternomastoid and left internal carotid arteries still measures 11 × 6 mm diameter is no longer FDG avid. No other pathologically enlarged cervical lymph node is seen and there is no pathologic FDG uptake in the neck.

There are a few tiny thyroid cysts bilaterally consistent with early multinodular goitre.

Thorax: The granulomata at the lung apices with adjacent fibrotic stranding and pleural thickening are unchanged. No pulmonary or mediastinal mass is seen and there is no pathologic FDG uptake.

Abdomen and Pelvis: The multiple hepatic cysts previously demonstrated are unchanged. Again here is no pathologic increased FDG uptake in the abdomen or pelvis.

This is an official medical report. If you are not the intended recipient, please contact our radiology practice immediately and advise us.

QUEENSLAND X-RAY PTY LTD ABN: XXXXX
XXXXXX Hospital Brisbane, SOUTH BRISBANE QLD 4101
Telephone: (07) 38406200 Facsimile: (07) 38461987

Calcified uterine fibroid noted on the left.

Musculoskeletal: The previously demonstrated foci of increased FDG uptake within mixed sclerotic and destructive lesions in the pelvis, sacrum, lumbothoracic and cervical spine are no longer FDG avid. No new skeletal lesions are detected.

Conclusion: Favourable response to therapy with diminished metabolic activity in widespread skeletal metastases, resolution of increased FDG uptake in a single left cervical lymph node level 2. No new metabolically active lesions.

DR: XXXXXXXXXXXXXXXXXXX
cc: DR XXXXXXXXXXXXXXXXXXXXX

This is an official medical report. If you are not the intended recipient, please contact our radiology practice immediately and advise us.

QUEENSLAND X-RAY PTY LTD ABN: XXXXX
Cairns XXXXXX, CAIRNS QLD 4870
Telephone: (07) 40467800 Facsimile: (07) 49467820

Monday, 15 November 2010
CAIRNS XXXXXX
CAIRNS QLD 4870

RE: **MRS DENICE JEFFERY** Patient ID:
Kewarra Beach QLD 4879
Service Date: 15/11/2010
Dept:
UR No:
Episode ID:

BONE MINERAL DENSITOMETRY

History: Ph mets breast cancer. On Arimidex. Exclude osteoporosis.

Procedure: Dual Energy X-Ray Absorptiometry (DEXA) of the lumbar spine and femoral neck.

Results: The average Bone Mineral Density of the lumbar spine (L2-4) is 1.16gm/cm^2 which is 106% of a young reference and lies 0.5 standard deviation above the mean for a young reference population (T-score). This is 0.87 standard deviations above the mean for aged matched control (Z-score).

The average BMD of the femoral neck is 0.89gm/cm^2 which is 95% of a young reference and lies 0.34 standard deviations below the mean for a young reference population (T-score). This is 0.35 standard deviations above the mean for aged matched control (Z-score).

Comment: These measurements are within normal limits and the fracture risk is not increased.

Thank you for referring this patient.

DR: XXXXXXXXXXXXXXXXXXXXXXXX
cc: XXXXXXXXXXXXXXXXXXXX

Printed in the USA
CPSIA information can be obtained
at www.ICGtesting.com
LVHW051620220624
783748LV00001B/207